Gout

Foods to Avoid

Foods to Enjoy

HR Research Alliance

This study aid is not intended to be any type of Medical advice. ALL individuals must consult their Doctors first and should always receive their meal plans from a qualified practitioner. This book is not intended to heal, or cure anyone from any kind of illness, or disease.

Table of Contents

Foods to Possibly Avoid: 9

Foods to Enjoy: 14

Butternut Beetroot Soup 20

Basil Avocado Zucchini Pasta 23

Spinach Coconut 26

Coconut Rice 29

Ginger and Coconut rice 32

Coconut Stuffed Avocado 35

Broccoli and Peanut Stir Fry 38

Coconut Currant Rice 41

Coconut Rice with Mango 44

Sweet and Sour Coconut Eggplant 47

Rosemary Potatoes 50

Vegan Basil Eggplant 52

Eggplant Chickpea Curry 56

Marinated Eggplant 59

Eggplant in Tomato Sauce 62

Roasted Eggplant Salad 65

Spicy Eggplant 69

Ginger Stir-Fry with Coconut Rice 73

Avocado Tacos 77

Lentil Bake 80

Tomato-Balsamic Veggies 84

Tempeh Fajitas 87

Red Turmeric Smoothie 91

Blueberry Cherry Blast 93

Sweet Cherry Greens 95

Red Creamy Honey Crisp 97

Ras-cherry 99

Cherry Mint Smoothie 101

Cherry Celery Smoothie 103

Papaya & Cherry 105

Mint Cherry Avo-Cacao 107

Gout is a type of arthritis. It is similar to, but different from rheumatoid arthritis.

Gout occurs when your body produces unusually high amounts of uric acid. Your kidneys may not excrete excess uric acid well and the levels rise in your blood. It is a severely painful type of arthritis, because excess uric acid forms into crystals. These crystals have a structure like needles and they "stab" into the joints and soft tissues of your body. Uric acid crystals irritate your tissues leading to inflammation and swelling.

Uric acid comes from purines in the diet.

A large number of people who suffer from gout tend to feel it in their big toe. In a smaller number of people, gout may affect other joints in the body such as your knees, wrists, elbows, ankles and fingers.

Over time, the uric acid crystals can build up near the joints and you will notice lumps under your skin. These are called, tophi. These crystals can also cause kidney stones. You can also develop "tophi" in your eyes, earlobes, soft tissues of the fingers, and even your lungs. One of the differences between rheumatoid arthritis and gout is that gout occurs in episodes. You may have a "gout flare up" that can last for a few days, all the way up to a few weeks. The symptoms can subside for a while and then come back. Rheumatoid arthritis is a chronic condition where some level of symptoms tend to be present at all times.

We are going share with you the variety of foods that you can eat with gout. And also we are going to share with you the other types of foods that you should avoid with gout. Each person has a unique circumstance when it comes to gout flare ups, and what foods trigger those flare ups.

It is always between you, and your qualified practitioner to decide which foods you personally can, and cannot consume. Some people with just minor gout flare ups, can consume even all of the foods on the avoid list. While others may still have to avoid foods on the enjoy list. These foods on each list have been researched, and are widely known for either their high, or low purine content. Not all foods high in purines will trigger gout pain for some individuals. And often times, it is more than the diet that is the cause of gout flare ups. Although it is always best to support a healthy lifestyle. And a diet low in processed foods, and high in fruits & vegetables, is a good place to begin the process towards healthy living. Keep these thoughts in your mind as you choose the perfect diet for your own needs.

Foods to Possibly Avoid:

Organ Meats (Liver, kidney, heart, brain, tongue, tripe).

- These are considered to have a high level of purines per serving, and should be avoided by most, and greatly reduced by others.

Wild Game (Venison, pheasant, veil, and more)

- All contain high levels of purines, and should be avoided by many gout sufferers.

Pork

- Known to be high in purines per serving. If eaten, one should reduce their consumption of pork to 4 oz. Or eliminate it completely from the diet.

Yeasts
- Known to trigger gout pain. Brewers yeast contains 1800 mg of purines in just 100 g serving.

Fish (Herring, mackerel, sardines, anchovies, & more)
- These fish contain the higher amounts of purines per serving. And should be avoided by most people with gout. More moderate amounts of purines in fish are in Salmon, Tuna, Codfish, Halibut, Snapper, & Trout. And still should be avoided by many with gout. And limited to just 4 oz by those who can consume them.

Shellfish (Oysters, scallops, shrimp, crab)
- These shellfish are all known to trigger gout pain. And contain high amounts of purines. Most who have gout should avoid all shellfish.

Whole Grains (Oatmeal, cereals, whole grain breads)

- While wholegrains can be consumed in moderation by many who have gout. They do contain higher levels of purines, and should be limited to small servings.

Refined Flours – White Breads – Pasta – White Rice

- All these foods should be avoided by many who have gout. For those who can consume these foods. They should limit them to small servings, not on a regular basis.

Alcohol

- Has been known to induce gout flair ups. Especially when drinking beer, which contains brewers yeast. Excessive alcohol consumption has been known to increase risk of gout attacks. 1 serving of wine is the best choice of alcohol for those with gout. Most should avoid alcohol completely. Especially beer.

Refined Sugars & High Fructose Corn Syrup

- Refined sugars themselves are low in purines. But a high refined sugar intake, has been linked to other conditions that can worsen gout flair ups. Avoid these for overall health.

Soft Drinks & Fruit Drinks

- Avoid these beverages. They contain high amounts of refined sugars, and high fructose corn syrup, which can worsen gout in many.

Meats – Turkey – Chicken

- Some Doctors may have a person avoid these completely. While others may have them consume them in moderation. The lower the fat content the better in these foods. Especially the saturated fat. And keep servings down to just a small portion. 4 oz.

Some vegetables such as asparagus, mushrooms, spinach, & cauliflower are higher in purines. Although they have not been found to worsen gout symptoms, or flare ups. Consume them in moderation of your Doctor has you do so.

Reducing fast foods, or eliminating them completely can have a great effect on your health. Many fast foods contain high amounts of the foods to avoid for gout. They should be avoided for overall health.

Foods to Enjoy:

Fresh Fruits

- Fruits are a great source of carbohydrates, without the refined sugars, high fructose corn syrup, and are low in purines. Making a wide variety of fruits a good choice for those with gout. Eat fruits high in vitamin C, such as oranges, tangerines, apples, avocados, & papaya.
- Dark cherries, and tart cherry extract, has been known to lower uric acid levels in the body. Many people with gout consume some sort of cherry each day. Whether they snack on them whole. Or, drink cherry extract juice. Cherry extract has been linked to 40% less risk of gout flare ups. Consider adding cherries, or cherry extract to your daily diet.

Vegetables
- A wide variety of vegetables are good for consumption with gout. One should consider adding several servings of mixed vegetables to their diet each day, for overall health.

Legumes
- For most people, beans, and lentils in moderation are fine. Reduce portion sizes if necessary. They contain moderate amounts of purines.

Nuts
- Many nuts are fine for those with gout. Good sources of nuts for gout are walnuts, almonds, & cashews.

Tubers

- All potatoes including sweet potato, contain low amounts of purines. Making them a great choice for gout. They also contain many nutrients promoting overall health.

Plant Based Oils

- Oils such as coconut oil, avocado oil, olive oil, and other plant based oils, are all fine for gout. And you can cook your foods using moderate amounts of them. Avoid genetically modified oils, such as canola oil.

Whole Grains

- These foods can be consumed in moderation by some who have gout. Others may need to avoid them, or reduce them to small portions.

Coffee & Tea

- In moderation, these are fine for gout. One should limit their caffeine consumption for overall health. 1, or 2 cups of coffee, or tea, is ok.

Eggs & Low Fat Dairy Products

- Eggs, and low fat dairy products, such as milk, cheese, and yogurt, are all good for gout. Consume them in your daily diet if desired.

Beef & Chicken

- High quality, hormone free beef, and chicken can be consumed in small portions. 4 oz. Choose low saturated fat cuts of these foods.

Herbs and spices

- Many herbs and spices are known for their aid in chronic inflammation in the body. And can be great for condiments on your meals. Spices such as turmeric, sage, cayenne pepper, rosemary, ginger, and cinnamon, can all be great for reducing inflammation. Making all spices a nice addition to cooked meals. And even to smoothies.

Tofu

- Tofu is preferred source of protein for those with gout. And can be consumed regularly. Use the recipes we provide for reference to making tofu dishes in your household.

Water

- Drinking plenty of water is beneficial for overall health. Staying hydrated during a gout attack can flush out uric acid crystals from the body.

It has been noted that following the Mediterranean diet, is the preferred choice of those with gout. The Mediterranean diet consists of many of the ingredients on the "enjoy" list. Others like to follow a more vegetarian, or vegan, plant based diet. All three choices are of the best for gout. Although, you and your Doctor will have to decide what is best for you. Many nutrients will be lacking in a vegan diet, that will have to be made up for with supplementation. In general, one should make an effort to eliminate processed, and refined foods from their diet. And replace them with whole foods, that are not man made. Next, we want to share some recipes with you, containing many of the ingredients in the "enjoy" category. Consider adding any of them into your diet. And discard the ones that do not fit into what you can eat. We provide a section for your notes, so you can create your own personal variation of the recipes provided.

Butternut Beetroot Soup

Ingredients:

- 1 Ounce of Coconut Oil
- 2 red Onions – Chopped
- 1 Butternut Squash
- 28 Ounces of Beetroot – Peeled, Chopped, Cooked
- 15 Ounces of Sweet Potato – Peeled, Chopped
- 10 Ounces of Leeks – Chopped
- 2 Cloves of Garlic – Minced
- 1 tsp. of Cinnamon
- 33 Ounces of vegetable Stock
- 1 tsp. of Nutmeg
- 1 inch Piece of Ginger – Peeled, Chopped
- Dash of Sea Salt
- Dash of Pepper
- Coriander – Chopped

Directions:

1. Sauté the onions, ginger, and the garlic for 3 minutes on medium heat.
2. Add in the leeks and stir it well for another 5 minutes.
3. Add in the squash, beetroot, and the sweet potatoes. Cover it with the stock.
4. Add in the cinnamon, salt, pepper, and the nutmeg. Stir it.
5. Bring it to a boil, cover it and allow it to simmer for 30-40 minutes until the vegetables are soft.
6. Stir in the chopped coriander and the chili flakes.

Nutritional Information per serving:

- Calories: 120
- Total Fat: 2g
- Saturated Fat: 1g
- Carbohydrates: 18g
- Protein: 3g

Notes

RECIPE

Variation ideas – Schedules - Notes

Basil Avocado Zucchini Pasta

Ingredients:

- 5 Small Zucchinis
- 3 Avocados
- ¾ Cup of Fresh Basil Leaves – Chopped
- 1 tsp. of Sea Salt
- 3 tsp. of Garlic Powder
- 3 Tbsp. of Extra Virgin Olive Oil
- ½ Lemon
- 2 Tbsp. of Coconut Oil
- 2 tsp. of Onion Powder
- 3 Strips of Cooked Tofu Bacon – Chopped

Directions:

1. Cut the zucchini into noodles.
2. Put the zucchini in your strainer.
3. Grind 4-5 twists of the sea salt on it.
4. Allow it to sit for 20 minutes.

5. Wrap the zucchini noodles in a cheesecloth or paper towels. Squeeze them gently. Put them aside.
6. Put the avocados, 1 tsp. of sea salt, basil, olive oil, garlic, and lemon juice in a food processor. Blend it until it is smooth.
7. Heat the coconut oil in a pan on medium heat.
8. Add in the zucchini noodles and the onion to sauté it for 2-3 minutes.
9. Add in the avocado sauce and toss it to coat it.
10. Stir it and top it with the bacon pieces.

Nutritional Information per serving:

- Calories: 470
- Total Fat: 22g
- Carbohydrates: 24g
- Protein: 17g

Notes

RECIPE

Variation ideas – Schedules - Notes

Spinach Coconut

Ingredients:

- Extra Virgin Olive Oil
- 2 Spring Onions – Sliced
- 2 Tbsp. of Curry Paste
- 17 Ounces of Tempeh chunks
- 13 Ounces of Pumpkin – Cut to Cubes
- 13 Ounces of Coconut Cream
- 13 Ounces of Fresh Spinach – Chopped

Directions:

1. Heat the oil in a large pan and cook it gently with the spring onions and the curry paste.
2. Add the tempeh and stir the chunks until it is browned.
3. Add in the coconut cream and the pumpkin cubes. Mix it gently.
4. Cover the pan with a lid and allow it to simmer on low for 20 minutes.

5. Stir it occasionally.
6. Before you serve it, add in the chopped spinach and stir it gently for 2-3 minutes.
7. Serve it with the coconut threads on the top.

Nutritional Information per serving:

- Calories: 460
- Total Fat: 15g
- Carbohydrates: 16g
- Protein: 28g

Notes

RECIPE

Variation ideas – Schedules - Notes

Coconut Rice

Ingredients:

- 1 Cup of Basmati Rice
- 14 Ounces of Coconut Milk – Light
- ¾ Cup of Water
- 1 Tbsp. of Virgin Coconut Oil
- 1 tsp. of Sea Salt
- 2 tsp. of Virgin Coconut Oil
- 2 Cloves of Garlic – Crushed
- 1 Red Chili Peppers – Finely Chopped
- 1 Medium Sized white Onion – Chopped
- 1 tsp. of Cumin Seed
- 1 Carrot – Chopped
- ½ Cup of Sweet Corn
- ½ Cup of Peas
- ½ Cup of Beansprouts
- ½ tsp. of Turmeric
- ½ tsp. of Coriander – Ground

- ½ tsp. Garam Masala
- 1 Tbsp. of Curry Powder
- 1 tsp. of Cumin
- ½ tsp. of Chilies – Puree
- Dash of Pepper

Directions:

1. Prepare the rice. Add the water, coconut milk, coconut oil, and the salt to a pan and bring it to a boil on medium heat.
2. Once it boils, add in the rice. Allow it to cook until it is done.
3. When the rice has 5 minutes left, add in the rest of the ingredients. Stir it all together.

Nutritional Information per serving:

- Calories: 410
- Total Fat: 15g
- Carbohydrates: 44g
- Protein: 6g

Notes

RECIPE

Variation ideas – Schedules - Notes

Ginger and Coconut rice

Ingredients:

- 2 Cups of vegetable Broth
- ½ Cup of Coconut Milk – Reduced Fat
- 2 tsp. of Ginger – Grated
- 1 Cup of Brown Rice – Uncooked
- ½ tsp. of Lemon Zest
- 2 Green Onions – Chopped
- 2 Tbsp. of Flaked Coconut – Toasted
- Lemon Slice for Garnishing (optional)

Directions:

1. Heat the broth, ginger, and coconut milk to a boil in a pan on medium high heat.
2. Stir in the rice.
3. Heat it to a boil and then reduce the heat.
4. Cover it and allow it to simmer for 15 minutes.
5. Add in the lemon zest and the green onions.

6. Fluff the rice with a fork.
7. Garnish it with coconut and the lemon slices.

Nutritional Information:

- Calories: 187
- Total Fat: 3g
- Carbohydrates: 28g
- Protein: 2g

Notes

RECIPE

Variation ideas – Schedules – Notes

Coconut Stuffed Avocado

Ingredients:

- 2 Ripened Avocado (Sliced and pitted.)
- 1 ½ Cups of Edamame – Shelled
- ½ Cup of Unsweetened Coconut – Toasted
- 2 Tbsp. of Diced Red Onion
- 2 Tbsp. of Parsley – Chopped
- 2 Tbsp. of Nori – Chopped
- 1 tsp. of Dijon Mustard
- 1 tsp. of Soy Sauce
- 3 Tbsp. of Lemon Juice
- 2 Tbsp. of Olive Oil
- Dash of Pepper
- Dash of Salt

Directions:

1. In a large mixing bowl, add in the edamame, coconut, red onion, parsley, and nori.
2. In a small mixing bowl, add in mustard, soy sauce, and the lemon juice.
3. Whisk the olive oil into the mustard mixture slowly. Add in the salt and pepper to taste.
4. Pour the filling into the avocado.

Nutritional Information per serving:

- Calories: 260
- Total Fat: 29g
- Saturated Fat: 7g
- Carbohydrates: 18g
- Protein: 8g

Notes

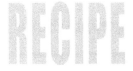

Variation ideas – Schedules - Notes

Broccoli and Peanut Stir Fry

Ingredients:

- 1 – 16 Ounce Package of Tofu – Firm
- 2 Cups of Uncooked Rice – Brown
- ½ tsp. of Sea Salt
- 1 ½ Cups of Vegetable Broth
- 2 Tbsp. of Lime Juice
- 2 Tbsp. of Chili Sauce – Sweet
- 2 Tbsp. of Peanut Butter – Creamy
- 1 Tbsp. of Soy Sauce – Lite
- 1 tsp. of Ginger
- 1 Tbsp. of Peanut Oil
- 2 Cups of Broccoli Florets
- 1 Cup of Carrot Sticks
- 2 Tbsp. of Peanuts – Chopped

Directions:
1. Put the tofu in between 2 flat plates.
2. Put a heavy can on top of the plates.

(The tofu should come out of the sides. Let it stand for 45 minutes).

3. Cut the tofu into half-inch cubes.
4. Cook the rice using the instructions on the package and add the salt.
5. In a medium-mixing bowl, add in the oil and tofu.
6. Add the vegetables and sauté them until they are browned; 10 minutes.
7. Add in the tofu and sauté for another 5 minutes.
8. Add the marinade and bring it to a boil or until it is thick.

Nutritional Information:
- Calories: 400
- Total Fat: 13g
- Carbohydrates: 58g
- Protein: 15g

Notes

RECIPE

Variation ideas – Schedules - Notes

Coconut Currant Rice

Ingredients:

- 1 Tbsp. of Olive Oil
- ½ Red Onion – Small, Finely Chopped
- 1 Clove of Garlic – Finely Chopped
- 1 Tbsp. of Grated Ginger
- 1 Cup of Basmati Rice
- 1 Cup of Light Coconut Milk
- 1 ½ Cups of Water

Directions:

1. Heat the oil in a 12-inch skillet on medium-high heat.
2. Cook the onion, ginger, garlic, and rice until the rice is finished according to directions.
3. Stir in the coconut milk.
4. Bring it to a boil on high heat.
5. Reduce the heat to medium and cook it for 5 minutes; stir it frequently.

6. Add the water and bring it to a boil again.
7. Reduce the heat to low and allow it to simmer for 10 minutes.
8. Reduce the heat to low and allow it to simmer (covered) for another 5 minutes.

Nutritional Information:

- Calories: 210
- Total Fat: 3g
- Carbohydrates: 27g
- Protein: 4g

Notes

RECIPE

Variation ideas – Schedules – Notes

Coconut Rice with Mango

Ingredients:

- 1 ½ Cups of Sticky Rice
- 1 Cup of Coconut Milk – Unsweetened
- ½ tsp. of Sea Salt
- 2 Mangos – Sliced
- 8 Mint Leaves – Garnish

Directions:

1. Put the sticky rice in a medium bowl and cover it with cold water. Allow it to soak overnight.
2. Drain the rice, place the rice in a microwave safe medium sized bowl.
3. Cover it with four cups of cold water.
4. Cover the bowl with a plate, and then microwave it for 3 minutes and stir.
5. Continue to microwave the rice and stir it every 3 minutes until the rice is fluffy. (10-12 minutes)
6. Put the coconut milk into a medium saucepan.

7. Turn the heat to medium and cook it until the milk is heated; yet not boiling.
8. Add the salt; stir it until it is dissolved.
9. Move the rice to a large mixing bowl.
10. Cover it with coconut milk and stir the rice until it begins to absorb the liquid. Let it stand for 1 hour.
11. Top the rice with pieces of the mango and garnish it with mint.

Nutritional Information:

- Calories: 320
- Total Fat: 5g
- Carbohydrates: 32g
- Protein: 7g

Notes

RECIPE

Variation ideas – Schedules – Notes

Sweet and Sour Coconut Eggplant

Ingredients

- 3 Tbsp. of Virgin Olive Oil – Cooking
- 2 Medium Sized Eggplants – Sliced to ½ Inch
- 2 Medium Sized Red Onion – ½ Inch Dice
- 3 Ribs of Celery – Cut into ½ inch pieces.
- 1 Cup of White Wine Vinegar
- 1/3 Cup of Coconut Flakes
- Dash of Salt
- Dash of Pepper

Directions:

1. In a large frying pan heat the oil.
2. Very carefully add the slices of eggplant; working in batches. Do not crowd the pan.
3. Cook the eggplant until it is gold on both sides. Place cooked pieces on a paper towel lined pan.
4. Add the celery and onions; sauté them until they are browned.

5. Remove it from the heat, and then add the vinegar, coconut flakes, salt, pepper.
6. Place the cooled off eggplant in a large mixing bowl. Cover it with the vinegar mix and allow it to stand for 1 hour.

Nutritional Information:

- Calories: 158
- Total Fat: 9g
- Carbohydrates: 13g
- Protein: 5g

Notes

RECIPE

Variation ideas – Schedules – Notes

Rosemary Potatoes

Ingredients:

8 Gold potatoes (sliced and quartered)

1 tbsp rosemary (dried)

¼ cup olive oil

Salt (to taste)

Black Pepper (to taste)

Directions:

Preheat the oven to 350 degrees F.

In a large bowl, combine the potatoes, oil and rosemary.

Season the potatoes with salt and pepper.

Spread the potatoes evenly on a cookie sheet and bake for approximately 30 minutes.

Nutrition information per serving:

- Calories 200
- Fats 3g
- Carbs 40g
- Pro 2g

Notes

Variation ideas – Schedules – Notes

Vegan Basil Eggplant

Ingredients:

- 1 large Italian eggplant, cut into 3/4 inch slices
- 4 tbsp coconut oil
- 2 garlic cloves, minced
- 14 oz firm tofu, block
- 1 red onion, sliced
- 1 green bell pepper, sliced
- 1 red bell pepper, sliced
- 1 yellow bell pepper, sliced
- Basil leaves
- For sauce:
- 2 tsp cornstarch
- 2 tsp chili sauce
- 1/4 cup water
- 1/2 cup tamari
- 4.5 tbsp Hoisin sauce

Directions:

1. Cut eggplant slices into 2 to 3 pieces each.
2. Heat 2 tbsp coconut oil in a pan over medium heat.
3. Add eggplant pieces into the pan and coat well with oil.
4. Add little water to the pan and cover and cook eggplant.
5. Stir eggplant pieces every few minutes.
6. Once the eggplant is cooked then turn off the heat and set pan aside.
7. Cut tofu into the pieces and squeeze out excess liquid from tofu.
8. Heat 1 tbsp oil in a pan over medium heat.
9. Add tofu to the pan and cook until golden brown.
10. Transfer cooked tofu to the eggplant pan.
11. Heat remaining oil in a pan and sauté bell peppers and onion and crispy. Add garlic and sauté for a minute.

12. Transfer onion and bell pepper mixture to the eggplant and tofu pan.

13. Whisk all sauce ingredients together.

14. Heat eggplant mixture pan over medium heat.

15. Once the pan is hot then add sauce mixture over veggies and mix well and cook for few minutes.

16. Remove pan from heat and add chopped basil.

17. Stir well and serve.

Nutritional Value (Amount per Serving):

- Calories 204
- Fat 12 g
- Carbohydrates 16 g
- Protein 9 g

Notes

RECIPE

Variation ideas – Schedules – Notes

Eggplant Chickpea Curry

Ingredients:

- 1 large eggplant, cut into pieces
- 15 oz can chickpeas, drained and rinsed
- 1/4 tsp cayenne pepper
- 1/4 tsp smoked paprika
- 1/4 tsp turmeric
- 1/2 tsp ground cumin
- 1 tsp onion powder
- 1 tbsp curry powder
- 1 cup coconut milk
- 2 garlic cloves, minced
- 1/2 red onion, diced
- Pepper
- Salt

Directions:

1. Add onion and eggplant into the large pan and cook over medium heat for 5 minutes. Add garlic and for a minute.
2. Add chickpea to the pan and stir well.
3. Add coconut milk, spices, pepper, and salt. Stir well and simmer for 5 minutes.
4. Stir well and serve.

Nutritional Value (Amount per Serving):

- Calories 321
- Fat 6 g
- Carbohydrates 55 g
- Protein 16 g

Notes

RECIPE

Variation ideas – Schedules – Notes

Marinated Eggplant

Ingredients:

- 2 large eggplant, cut into 1/4 inch slices
- 1 tbsp vinegar
- 4.5 tbsp olive oil
- 2 garlic cloves, chopped
- 1/4 cup fresh mint, chopped
- 1 tbsp oregano
- 1/2 red chili
- Salt

Directions:

1. Add sliced eggplant into the mixing bowl.
2. Sprinkle a little salt over the slices eggplant and set aside for 30 minutes to release some water.
3. Rinse eggplant well and pat dry with paper towel.
4. Brush eggplant with oil.
5. Place eggplant slices on the hot griddle pan and cook until softened.

6. In a small bowl, mix together all remaining ingredients and set aside.
7. Arrange cooked eggplant slices on serving dish and drizzle marinade over the eggplant slices.
8. Serve and enjoy.

Nutritional Value (Amount per Serving):

- Calories 134
- Fat 10 g
- Carbohydrates 10 g
- Protein 1 g

Notes

RECIPE

Variation ideas – Schedules – Notes

Eggplant in Tomato Sauce

Ingredients:

- 1 medium eggplant, cut into cubes
- 3 golden potatoes, boiled and cut into cubes
- 14 oz can tomatoes, crushed
- 1 tbsp curry powder
- 6 garlic cloves, chopped
- 2 tbsp olive oil
- 1 tsp salt

Directions:

1. Heat olive oil in the pan over medium heat.
2. Add eggplant cubes to the pan and cook for few minutes.
3. Add curry powder, garlic, and salt and cook for a minute.
4. Add crushed tomatoes and stir well and simmer for 5 minutes.

5. Add potato cubes and cook for a minute.
6. Stir well and serve.

Nutritional Value (Amount per Serving):

- Calories 232
- Fat 7 g
- Carbohydrates 39 g
- Protein 5 g

Notes

RECIPE

Variation ideas – Schedules - Notes

Roasted Eggplant Salad

Ingredients:

- 2 large eggplants, cut in half then sliced
- 1 tbsp olive oil
- 1/4 cup basil leaves, chopped
- 3/4 cup cilantro, chopped
- 1 lemon juice
- 3 tomatoes
- 1 green bell pepper, cut in half and remove seeds
- 1 yellow bell pepper, cut in half and remove seeds
- 1 red bell pepper, cut in half and remove seeds
- Salt

Directions:

1. Place sliced eggplant into the bowl and sprinkle with salt. Set aside for 30 minutes.
2. After 30 minutes rinse the sliced eggplants and pat dry with paper towel.
3. Preheat the oven to 350 F.
4. Spray a baking tray with cooking spray.
5. Place sliced eggplant on prepared baking tray and roast in preheated oven for 10 minutes.
6. Place tomatoes and bell pepper on another baking tray and roast for 50 minutes.
7. Remove eggplant. bell pepper, and tomatoes from oven and set aside to cool.
8. Once veggies are cool then scrap eggplant flesh onto a cutting board and cut into pieces.
9. Remove skin and seed of tomatoes and cut into pieces.
10. Remove the skin of bell pepper and cut bell pepper into the pieces.

11. Add chopped eggplant, bell pepper, and tomatoes into the large mixing bowl.

12. Add remaining ingredients into the bowl and toss well.

13. Serve and enjoy.

Nutritional Value (Amount per Serving):

- Calories 147
- Fat 4 g
- Carbohydrates 26 g
- Protein 4 g

Notes

Variation ideas – Schedules - Notes

Spicy Eggplant

Ingredients:

- 3 medium eggplants, sliced into wedges
- 1/2 cup basil, chopped
- 4 green onions, chopped
- 2 bell pepper, cut into strips
- 8 oz mushrooms, sliced
- 2 tbsp coconut oil
- 1 tbsp salt
- For sauce:
- 1/4 cup vegetable broth
- 1 tbsp rice vinegar
- 1 tbsp soy sauce
- 2 tbsp tamari
- 3 tsp sesame oil
- 1/4 cup brown sugar (optional)
- 1/4 cup sweet chili sauce
- 2 tbsp chili paste

- 3 garlic cloves, minced

Directions:

1. Add eggplant into the bowl and sprinkle salt over the eggplant and set aside for 15 minutes.
2. Rinse eggplant slices and pat dry with paper towel.
3. In a bowl, whisk all sauce ingredients together.
4. Melt coconut oil in the pan over medium-high heat.
5. Add eggplant and cook until it is tender.
6. Remove eggplant from pan and place on a plate.
7. Add green onion, mushrooms, and bell peppers into the pan and sauté for 5 minutes.
8. Add eggplant and sauce. Let simmer for 10 minutes.
9. Add basil and stir well.
10. Serve and enjoy.

Nutritional Value (Amount per Serving):

- Calories 333
- Fat 12 g
- Carbohydrates 51 g
- Protein 8 g

Notes

RECIPE

Variation ideas – Schedules - Notes

Ginger Stir-Fry with Coconut Rice

Ingredients:

- 1/2 clove garlic, crushed
- 1/2 tsp. chopped fresh ginger root, divided
- 2 tsp. extra virgin olive-oil, divided
- 1/4 cup broccoli florets
- 1 Tbsp. snow peas
- 2 Tbsp. julienned carrots
- 1 Tbsp. red bell pepper, diced
- 1 tsp. soy sauce
- 1 tsp. water
- 1/2 Tbsp. chopped onion
- 1/4 cup jasmine rice
- 1/4 cup coconut milk
- 1/4 cup water
- Sriracha (or other hot sauce)

Directions:

1. First prepare the rice by placing the rice, coconut milk, and water in a medium saucepan or small pot. Turn the heat to high until it begins to boil, and then reduce to low, cover and let simmer for 15 minutes, or until most of the coconut milk has been absorbed.

2. In a large bowl, blend garlic, half the ginger, and 1 tsp. olive oil.

3. Add the broccoli, snow peas, carrots, and bell pepper, tossing to lighting coat.

4. Heat the remaining olive oil in a wok over medium heat. Add vegetables, cook for 1 minute, stirring constantly to prevent burning.

5. Add onions, salt, remaining ginger, soy sauce and water. Cook until vegetables are tender, but still crisp— about 2 minutes.

6. Place coconut rice in a bowl, top with ginger stir fry. Add Sriracha to taste.

Nutritional Information

- **Calories: 338**
- **Total Fat: 16 g**
- **Carbohydrates: 42 g**
- **Protein: 6 g**

Notes

Variation ideas – Schedules – Notes

Avocado Tacos

Ingredients:

- 1 avocado, peeled, pitted, and mashed
- 2 Tbsp. onions, diced
- 1/8 tsp. garlic salt
- 1 tsp. lemon juice
- Drizzle olive oil
- 2 Tbsp. tomato, diced
- 2 tsp. cilantro, chopped
- 1/4 cup black beans, canned, drained and rinsed
- 1/2 garlic clove, chopped
- Salt and pepper, to taste

Directions:

1. Preheat oven to 325 degrees F.
2. In a medium saucepan, heat olive oil over medium heat and add the garlic and half the onions and cook until translucent, about 2-5 minutes.

3. Add the black beans, turn heat the low. Stir occasionally and allow the beans to heat while you work on the filling.

4. Arrange corn tortillas in a single layer on a large baking sheet, and place in the preheated oven 2 to 5 minutes, until heated through.

5. In a medium bowl, mix avocado, remaining onion, tomatoes, garlic salt, pepper, lemon juice and a drizzle of olive oil.

6. Spread tortillas with avocado mixture, add black beans and top with cilantro.

Nutritional Information

- **Calories: 377**
- **Total Fat: 18g**
- **Carbohydrates: 43 g**
- **Protein: 9g**

Notes

RECIPE

Variation ideas – Schedules – Notes

Lentil Bake

Ingredients:

- ½ cup long-grain rice, uncooked
- 2 ½ cups water
- 1 cup red lentils
- 1 tsp. coconut oil
- 1 small red onion, diced
- 3 cloves garlic, minced
- 1 tomato, diced
- 1/3 cup diced celery
- 1/3 cup chopped carrots
- 1/3 cup chopped green zucchini
- 1 (8 oz.) can tomato sauce
- 1 tsp. dried basil
- 1 tsp. dried oregano
- 1 tsp. ground cumin
- ½ tsp. celery seed
- Salt and pepper, to taste

Directions:

1. Preheat oven to 350 degrees F. In a small bowl, combine basil, oregano, cumin, celery seed, and a pinch of salt and pepper. Set aside.

2. Place the rice and 1 cup water in a medium pot over high heat and bring to a boil. Cover, reduce heat to low, and simmer 20 minutes.

3. Place lentils in a pot with the remaining 1 ½ cups water, and bring to a boil. Cook 15 minutes, or until tender.

4. Heat the oil in a skillet over medium heat, and stir in the onion and garlic. Mix in tomato, celery, carrots, zucchini, and ½ the tomato sauce. Season with ½ the seasoning mix.

5. In a casserole dish, mix the rice, lentils, and vegetables. Top with remaining tomato sauce, and sprinkle with remaining seasoning.

6. Bake 30 minutes in the preheated oven, until the top is bubbling. Remove and serve. Store leftovers in an airtight container, in the fridge, for up to a week.

Nutritional Information (for 1/6th of bake)

- **Calories: 192**
- **Total Fat: 1 g**
- **Carbohydrates: 35 g**
- **Protein: 9g**

Notes

RECIPE

Variation ideas – Schedules - Notes

Tomato-Balsamic Veggies

Ingredients:

- 1 tsp. olive oil
- ¼ red bell pepper, cut into strips
- 1 green zucchini, cut into thick slices
- ¼ small eggplant, cubed
- ¼ large sweet onion, diced
- ¼ cup frozen broad beans
- 2 tomatoes, diced
- 2 tsp. balsamic vinegar
- ¼ cup couscous
- ¼ cup vegetable stock

Directions:

1. Heat olive oil in a medium grill pan over high heat. When it is very hot, add all the vegetables to the pan. Press down occasionally to get grill lines across them. Turn occasionally to prevent burning. Cook for about 15 minutes, or until the vegetables are evenly browned and cooked through.

2. Add broad beans to the vegetables. Add diced tomatoes and balsamic vinegar. Simmer for a few minutes while you prepare the couscous.

3. Place couscous into a medium bowl. Add boiling vegetable stock, and stir with a fork. Cover and allow 2-3 minutes to become softened. Place couscous in a bowl and top with the vegetables.

Nutritional Information

- **Calories: 82**
- **Total Fat: 1 g**
- **Carbohydrates: 14 g**
- **Protein: 2 g**

Notes

RECIPE

Variation ideas – Schedules - Notes

Tempeh Fajitas

Ingredients:

- 1 ½ tsp. olive oil
- ¼ (8 oz.) package tempeh, broken into bite-size pieces
- 2 tsp. soy sauce
- 1 tsp. lime juice
- 1/2 chopped white onion
- 1 clove garlic, minced
- 1/3 cup chopped green bell pepper
- ¾ tsp. chopped green chile peppers
- 1 Tbsp. chopped fresh cilantro
- 2 corn tortillas

Directions:

1. Preheat oven to 350 degrees F.
2. Heat oil in medium skillet over medium heat. Add onion and garlic and cook for 3-5 minutes. Add tempeh with soy sauce and lime juice until tempeh browns.

3. Add bell peppers, chile peppers, and cilantro and turn heat to medium-high and cook for 5-10 minutes, stirring occasionally.

4. Meanwhile, heat the corn tortillas in preheated oven until warm and pliable, about 3-5 minutes.

5. Remove tortillas from oven, fill with tempeh mixture and enjoy.

Nutritional Information

- **Calories: 154**
- **Total Fat: 4 g**
- **Carbohydrates: 23 g**
- **Protein: 5.g**

Notes

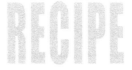

Variation ideas – Schedules - Notes

Smoothie recipes are an easy way to eat healthy. You can create them with a wide variety of gout friendly fruits, vegetables, and spices. Try these out, and create your own delicious smoothie recipes with gout friendly ingredients.

Red Turmeric Smoothie

Ingredients

- 1 cup dark cherries (frozen)
- ½ cup pineapple chunks
- ½ tsp. ground turmeric
- ½ cup tart cherry juice
- 4-6 ice cubes

Directions

1. Combine ingredients in a blender. Cover and blend until smooth.
2. Serve & enjoy!

Nutritional Information (per serving)

- Calories 222
- Fat 0 g
- Carbohydrates 55 g
- Protein 4 g

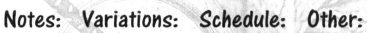

Notes: Variations: Schedule: Other:

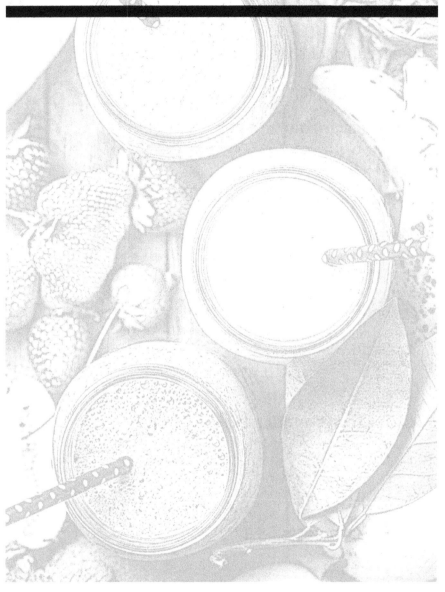

Blueberry Cherry Blast

Ingredients

- 1 pear, cored and chopped, with skin
- 1 cup dark cherries
- 1 cup frozen blueberries, unsweetened
- ½ tsp. cinnamon
- ½ cup coconut water
- 4 ice cubes

Directions

1. Combine ingredients in a blender. Cover and blend until smooth.
2. Serve & enjoy!

Nutritional Information (per serving)

- Calories 276
- Fat 1 g
- Carbohydrates 54 g
- Protein 2g

Notes: Variations: Schedule: Other:

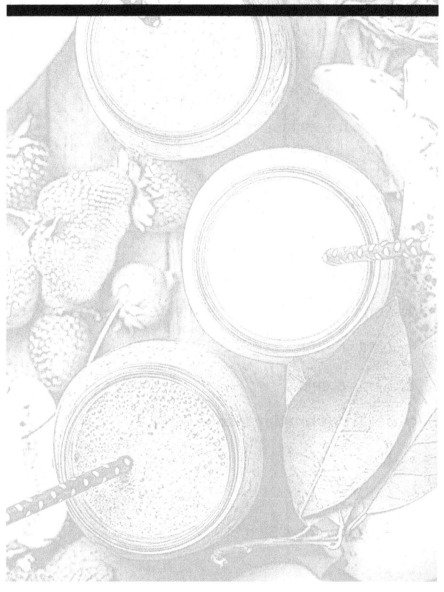

Sweet Cherry Greens

Ingredients

- 1 cup strawberries, halved
- 1 cup frozen black cherries, pitted
- 1 cup coconut water
- ½ cup green cabbage
- ½ cup green kale
- 3-6 ice cubes

*Optional ½ cup vanilla yogurt(or vegan)

Directions

1. Combine ingredients in a blender. Cover and blend until smooth.
2. Serve & enjoy!

Nutritional Information (per serving)

- Calories 237
- Fat 3 g
- Carbohydrates 54 g
- Protein 4 g

Notes: Variations: Schedule: Other:

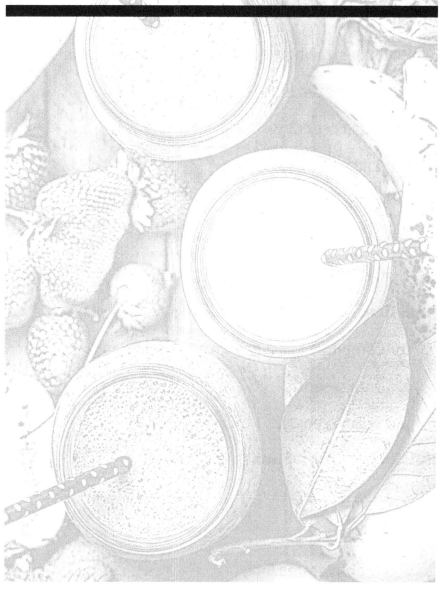

Red Creamy Honey Crisp

Ingredients

- 2 honey crisp apples, cored and quartered, with skin
- 2 tbsp. creamy almond butter
- 1/2 cup tart cherry juice
- ½ tsp. cinnamon
- ¼ tsp. nutmeg
- ½ inch fresh ginger

Directions

1. Combine ingredients in a blender. Cover and blend until smooth.
2. Serve & enjoy!

Nutritional Information (per serving)

- Calories 424
- Fat 20 g
- Carbohydrates 65 g
- Protein 10 g

Notes: Variations: Schedule: Other:

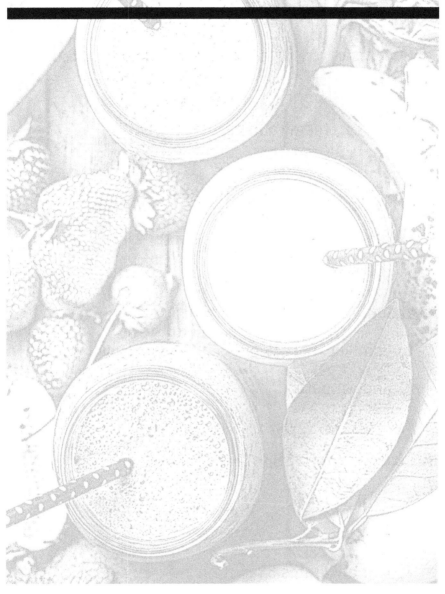

Ras-cherry

Ingredients

- 1 cup frozen cherries
- 1 cup frozen strawberries, unsweetened
- 1 small banana, peeled
- ½ cup red raspberries
- ¾ cup water
- 4 ice cubes

Directions

1. Combine ingredients in a blender. Cover and blend until smooth.
2. Serve & enjoy!

Nutritional Information (per serving)

- Calories 226
- Fat 1 g
- Carbohydrates 45 g
- Protein 2 g

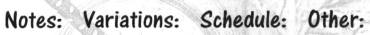

Notes: Variations: Schedule: Other:

Cherry Mint Smoothie

Ingredients:

- 2 ripe bananas
- 2 cups fresh cherries pitted
- 1/2 cup water
- 4 mint leaves
- 6 ice cubes
- Coconut flakes – not blended, on top

Directions:

1. Add all ingredients into the blender and blend until smooth.
2. Serve & enjoy!

Nutritional Value (Amount per Serving):

- Calories 247
- Fat 3 g
- Carbohydrates 50 g
- Protein 2 g

Notes: Variations: Schedule: Other:

Cherry Celery Smoothie

Ingredients

- 1 cup dark cherries
- 2 celery stalks, chopped
- ¾ cup tart cherry juice
- 1 tsp. lemon juice
- Pinch of cayenne pepper(optional)
- 4-6 ice cubes

Directions

1. Combine ingredients in a blender. Cover and blend until smooth.
2. Optional: pour and garnish with celery sticks.

Nutritional Information (per serving)

- Calories 85
- Fat 0 g
- Carbohydrates 24 g
- Protein 1 g

Notes: Variations: Schedule: Other:

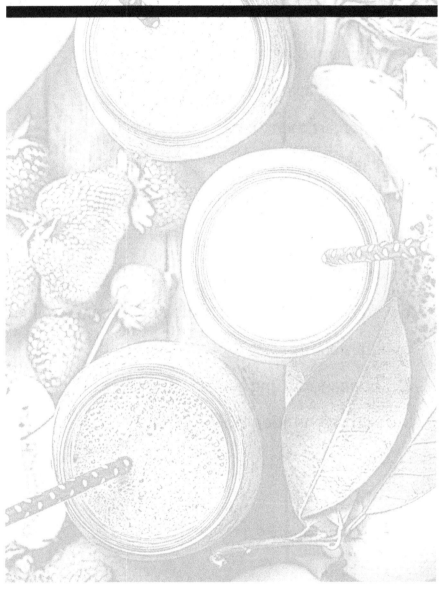

Papaya & Cherry

Ingredients

- 1 cup papaya, seeded and peeled
- 1 small banana, peeled
- ½ cup dark cherries
- 1 cup coconut water
- 4-6 ice cubes
- Optional: 1-2 dates for a sweeter smoothie

Directions

1. Combine papaya and water first. Cover and blend until smooth.
2. Serve & enjoy!

Nutritional Information (per serving)

- Calories 167
- Fat 1 g
- Carbohydrates 34 g
- Protein 2 g

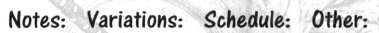

Notes: Variations: Schedule: Other:

Mint Cherry Avo-Cacao

Ingredients

- 1 avocado, pitted
- 2 ½ tbsp. raw cacao powder
- 1 banana, peeled
- 1 cup fresh cherries
- 3 tbsp. creamy peanut butter
- ¼ cup vanilla almond milk, unsweetened
- 1 lime – juice
- 4 mint leaves
- 3-4 ice cubes

Directions

1. Combine ingredients in a blender. Cover and blend until smooth.
2. Serve & enjoy!

Nutritional Information (per serving)

- Calories 586
- Fat 30 g   Carbohydrates 60 g   Protein 18 g

Notes: Variations: Schedule: Other:

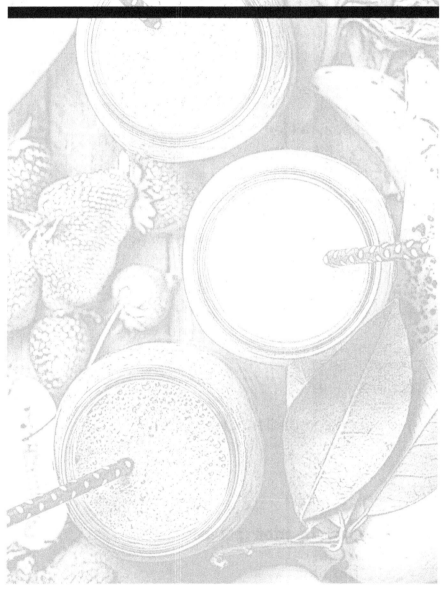

Join the free Gout & Inflammation Newsletter. Clickable links are inside of the eBook version of this book. Or, you can also email **goutinflammationinfo@gmail.com** and request the link to be sent to your email.

Text Copyright ©

All rights reserved. No part of this guide may be reproduced in any form without permission in writing from the publisher except in the case of brief quotations embodied in critical articles or reviews.

Legal & Disclaimer

The information contained in this book and its contents is not designed to replace or take the place of any form of medical or professional advice; and is not meant to replace the need for independent medical, or other professional advice or services. The content and information in this book has been provided for educational and entertainment purposes only.

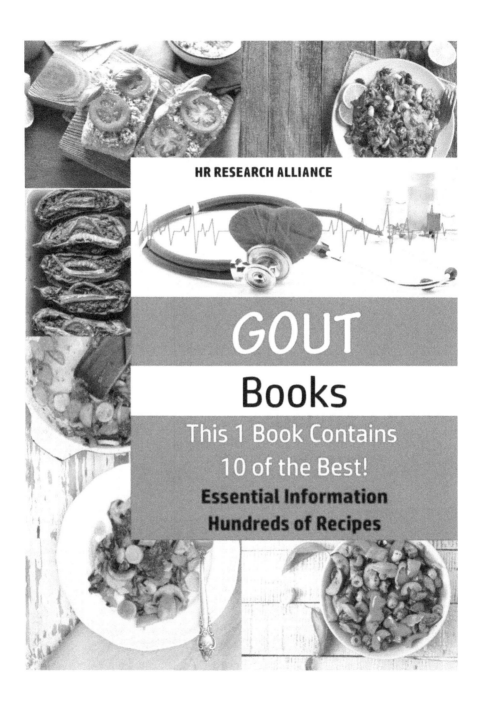

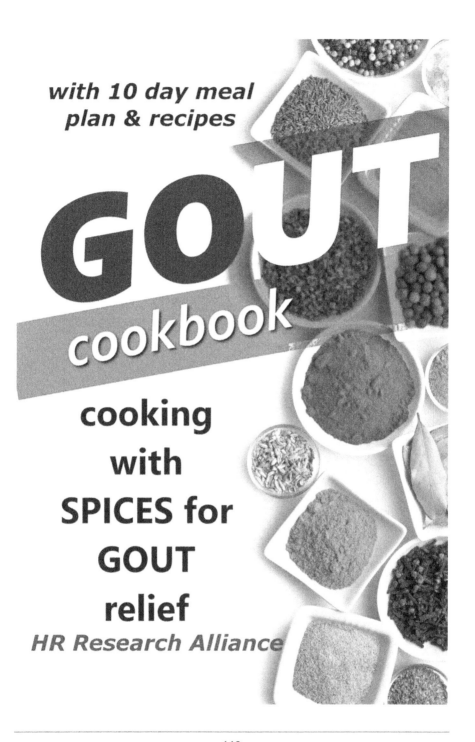

GOUT cookbook

with 10 day meal plan & recipes

cooking with SPICES for GOUT relief

HR Research Alliance

GOUT
Prevention

a metabolic disorder
uric acid

the deposition and accumulation
of salts in the joint

GOUT

inflammation and pain
in the small joints

Geoff Andersen

With Meal Plan & Gout Recipes

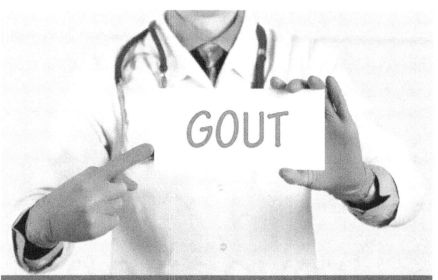

ANTI - INFLAMMATION
The Essential Gout & Arthritis Meal Plan Guide

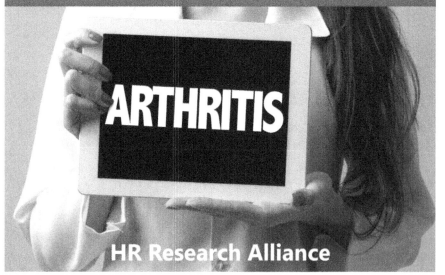

HR Research Alliance

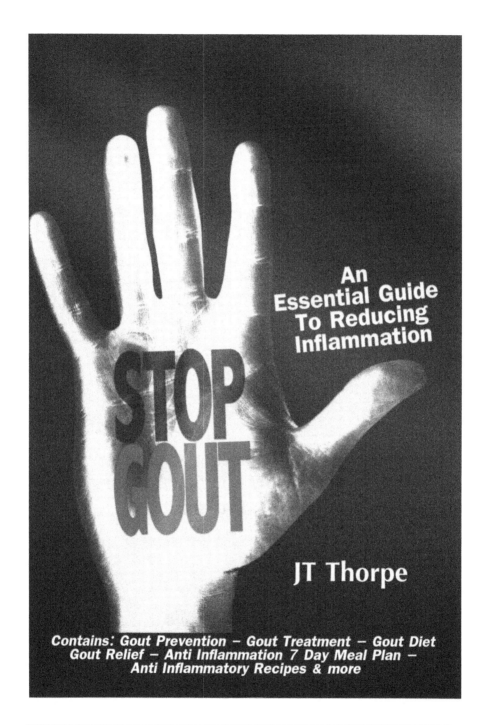

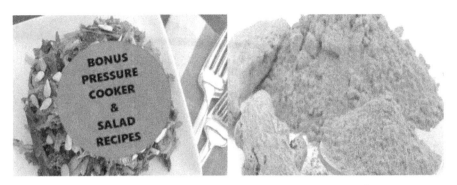

ANTI - INFLAMMATORY
COOKBOOK

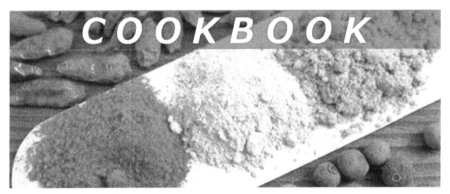

50 Slow Cooker Recipes With Anti - Inflammatory Ingredients

GREAT FOR GOUT RELIEF!

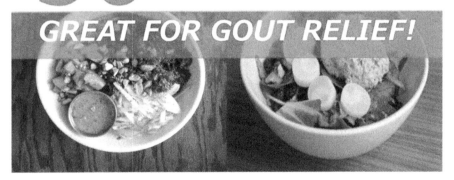

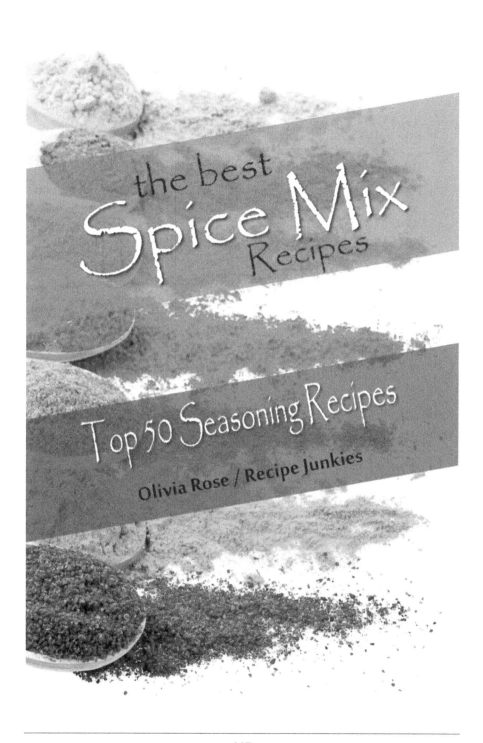

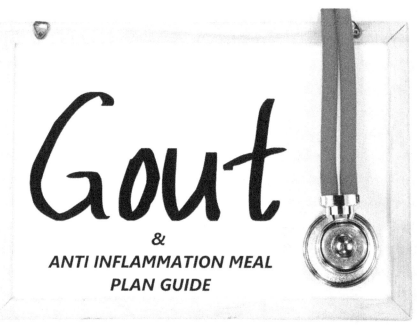

Gout
& ANTI INFLAMMATION MEAL PLAN GUIDE

Nutritional Strategies For Reducing Inflammation Naturally

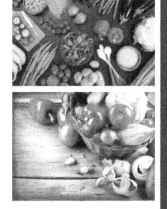

Gout Prevention - Gout Diet - Anti Inflammatory Foods To Eat & Avoid - & More...

HR Research Alliance

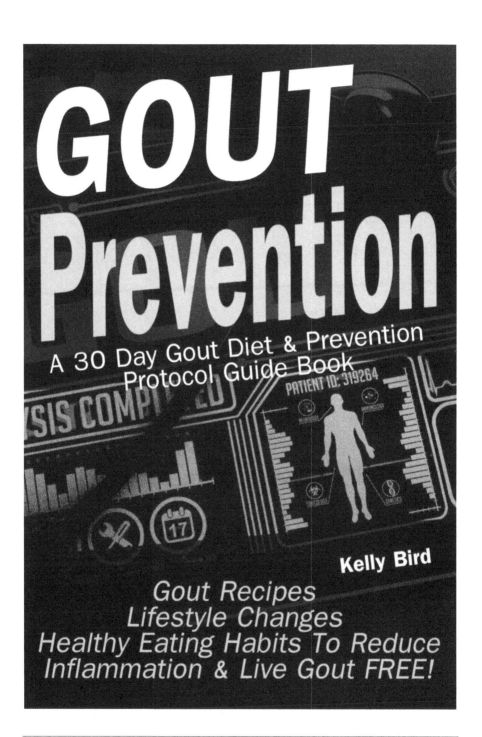

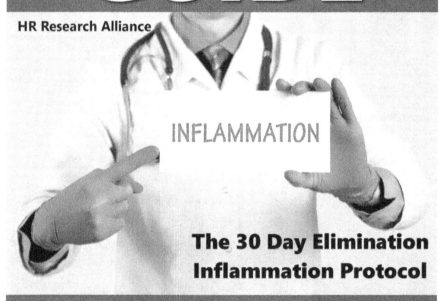

Made in the USA
Las Vegas, NV
04 May 2021